FROM Stress TO Profit

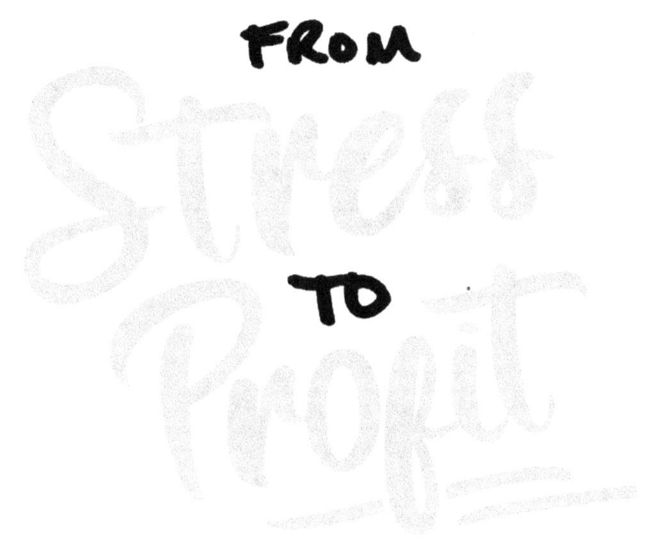

—— ADAM WEBER ——

There always seems to be a stress tsunami going on,
and you face an unprecedent amount of stress daily.

This book is dedicated to you, the corporate warrior
who faces stress day after day.

CONTENTS

Introduction..11

Our Stress-Filled Lives.............................. 15

The Modern Stress Epidemic 19

Stress and the Workplace........................... 23

Workplace Stress and Productivity Losses........... 27

Respond to Your Stress 31

The Stress Solution.................................... 35

What is Meditation? 37

Why you should meditate........................... 39

Meditation Myths and Truths.....................47

The Truth About Easy to Meditate....................51

When Should You Meditate? 53

How to Meditate 55

Creating Your Meditation Habit 61

Frequently Asked Questions 65

What to Expect with Easy to Meditate?............... 71

Staying Motivated to Meditate........................... 73

Conclusion 75

Bonus Chapters.................................... 81

Work with Adam.................................. 105

About Adam Weber 107

WORK WITH ADAM

There are five easy ways to work with Adam. The following five options are available based on your needs.

1. Read this short book, and then figure it out on your own.

2. Visit www.EasyToMeditate.com, read/watch the blog/vlog, and then figure it out on your own.

3. Invest in the Easy to Meditate online program.

4. Bring Adam into your business for training, coaching and get a special online program and video coaching after the training.

5. Custom training by design, based on your organization's needs.

Please visit www.EasyToMeditate.com for lots of bonuses and so that we can decide if working together is a good fit.

INTRODUCTION

My days in the corporate world usually started at 3:00 am when it was still dark outside, and I was wide awake.

Day after day, weekends too, it was like putting my foot on the gas pedal and not being able to find the brake to slow down or stop.

My body would ache to go back to sleep for just 15 more minutes.

But no, I was wide awake and the anticipation of a full day, being pulled in different directions with lots of stress was upon me.

I was working in commercial real estate for one of the world's corporate real estate giants.

And commercial real estate in New York City is well known for serving up stress on a silver platter.

And while I made great money. I let the work own me.

The stress was overwhelming.

I would blame my co-workers; I would blame the clients or some days I would blame my boss.

There were days that I would not eat, and there were nights that I could not sleep.

The stress was eating me alive and I was hurting.

I regularly became easily agitated, frustrated, and moody. I felt overwhelmed and felt like I was are losing control. I had difficulty relaxing.

I felt lonely, worthless, and depressed.

I avoided others like they were the plague, including those closest to me.

I swallowed my pride and scheduled an appointment with my doctor.

As if the stressful work wasn't enough, I was diagnosed with Primary Progressive Multiple Sclerosis.

Multiple Sclerosis is an incurable and debilitating disease. It is a life sentence.

The compound effect of my stressors was crazy.

I knew that I needed to make a change and tame my stress.

So, after speaking with my doctors and conducting exhaustive research I had an aha moment. A breakthrough moment.

My breakthrough. Meditation!

With meditation you can reduce your stress and calm your mind. The benefits are amazing.

My goal is to teach you an easy way, a clear path so that in just minutes a day you have a way to reduce your stress and to start living a happier and healthier life utilizing a technique that I developed called Easy to Meditate.

I teach this method because it is so powerful and when you empower yourself with a simple tool, like Easy to Meditate to deal with your stress, you are setting yourself up to win.

Easy to Meditate is an easy, simple, repeatable and effective meditation technique that can have a profound effect on your mind, your body and virtually every aspect of your life

When you find positive ways to deal with your stress, you are better prepared for your challenges.

OUR STRESS-FILLED LIVES

Do you suffer because of your stress?

Every day corporate warriors experience a tsunami of stress.

Stress is one of the most common health conditions today, and it accounts for millions of lost working days. Those lost days translate into billions of lost dollars.

Millions are suffering, but the good news is that the suffering can end.

Stress affects our home lives.

Stress affects our work lives.

And stress affects our health.

It does not matter who you are. It does not matter where you live. Stress does not care about your age or your net worth.

There is nothing worse than walking through your own big, dark and violent internal stress tsunami.

The June 6, 1983 *Time* magazine's cover story called stress "The Epidemic of the Eighties" and referred to it at the time as our leading health problem.

A 1996 survey from *Prevention* magazine found that approximately 75% of people feel that they have "great stress" one day a week, with 1 out of 3 indicating they feel this way more than twice a week.

So, what has changed?

Today Americans believe that they are under as much or even more stress than in the past.

It is estimated that approximately 75% of all our visits to our primary care doctors are for our stress-related problems.

Today, the situation has gotten much worse and job stress is the leading source of stress for adults.

The old model of fixing your stress, by just going to a doctor and getting a pill and hoping that the stress will go away, is a broken model.

At times, we all have intense and overwhelming stress tsunamis.

The onslaught of today's stress tsunamis includes both our personal and professional stress.

I want to ask you again: Have you ever thought about how you could reduce your stress?

By empowering yourself to deal with your stress, you are addressing your own self-care and refusing to lose to our stress.

By empowering yourself with a positive tool to deal with your stress, you are setting yourself up with a tool to maintain your own health and wellbeing.

Refuse to lose to your stress.

Research has revealed that if you take the time to manage and work to eliminate your stress that you can benefit on both a short-term and a long-term basis.

That is easier said than done.

You must take the necessary steps to reduce your bad stress and repeat these steps daily.

My goal is to show you an easy way, a clear path in just minutes a day, to reduce your stress and to start living a happier and healthier life.

That way is meditation. More specifically a technique that I developed called Easy to Meditate.

Easy to Meditate is a simple and easy-to- learn, step-by-step meditation technique that can be utilized to help reduce your stress.

By empowering yourself with a simple tool, like Easy to Meditate to deal with your stress, you are setting yourself up to win.

Studies have shown that a regular meditation practice can significantly reduce your stress, as well as tension, anxiety, depression, anger, hostility and fatigue.

This book will show you a simple, repeatable and effective way to deal with your stress utilizing meditation.

Easy to Meditate can have a profound effect on your body, your mind and virtually every aspect of your life

When you find a positive way to deal with your stress, you are better prepared for your challenges.

THE MODERN STRESS EPIDEMIC

Stress affects every aspects of your life and it is only getting worse.

Stress wears you down and makes you sick, both mentally and physically. No part of your body is immune.

When you are stressed, your body releases the "stress hormone" called cortisol, and elevated levels of cortisol in your system are a problem.

Finding a way to reduce your cortisol levels will help prevent several health issues from developing.

Chronic stress and prolonged chronic stress do not let up, and they should terrify you because they exact a toxic and harmful toll on your body, your brain, your mind and your soul.

You cannot always stop your stressors, but you can control how you respond to them.

The wellness publication, Everyday Health, surveyed 6,700 Americans with ages ranging from 18 to 64. The key takeaways from the survey were:

Chronic stress is a national epidemic for men and women between 25 to 35 years old.

Of those surveyed, approximately 1/3 say they have visited a doctor about their stress.

Of the survey respondents, 57% say they feel paralyzed by their stress, and 43% say they are invigorated by their stress.

51% of the women surveyed say they don't see friends at all in an average week.

59% of baby boomers have never been diagnosed with a mental health issue.

52% of Generation Z already have been diagnosed with a mental health issue.

Over a 33% of all men and women say that their work is a regular source of their stress.

Over 44% of those that are part of Generation Z say that their work is a regular source of their stress.

More than 51% of the women surveyed say they feel bad about their appearance weekly, and 28% say that their appearance regularly causes them stress. Only 34% of men say they feel bad about their appearance weekly.

52% say financial issues regularly stress them out. 35% cited jobs and careers as the next most common stressor.

47% equally weighted, between both women and men say that their response to stress is to take it out on themselves.

The most important takeaway was that stress is a national epidemic.

According to a recently completed poll of more than 2,000 Americans whose ages ranged from 22 to 37, the following are the top 15 reasons that both men and women feel stress.

1. Losing a wallet or a credit card

2. Arguing with a significant other

3. Their daily commute

4. Losing their mobile phone

5. Being late to work

6. Slow internet or WIFI

7. Their mobile phone's battery dying

8. Breaking their cell phone screen

9. Forgetting or losing passwords

10. The fraudulent use of their credit card

11. Credit card bills

12. Losing or forgetting their cell phone charger

13. Losing or misplacing their keys

14. Having to pay their bills

15. Interviewing for a job

The above reasons are real, and you need help dealing with your stress.

STRESS AND THE WORKPLACE

Jeff Bezos of Amazon does not believe in the term "work-life balance". As was cited in the magazine *Business Insider,* he refers to "work-life balance" as a "debilitating phrase" and the term "work-life balance" assumes a tradeoff.

When you are happier at home, you can perform better at work, and when you are happy at work, you can be more present at home.

The problem is that many of us do not feel that we are in control of own lives but rather we are beholden to the demands of our employer.

Is that you?

Having worked in the corporate world for more than 20 years, and having done extensive research, I can personally say that stress levels remain very high today.

That includes working long days, and for some the more-than-occasional all-nighter.

Too many experience, the draining effects of stress both at work and at home.

The 9-5 work schedule is a relic of the past, and anyone who attempts to work those hours is sometimes ridiculed as only working a half day at times.

Employees need to show that they are putting in the time , whether they are working or not, and long working hours has become synonymous with a successful career. The two are rarely stripped apart.

Longer hours and fewer days off have become the expectation of many employers, and employees are willingly putting in the long hours in order to stand out.

Is that you?

The remote work culture has only made the problem worse.

Today, work extends far beyond the office with many working late during the week, working on weekends and even working while on vacation.

This should not be new if you work in the corporate world today. Either you, your coworkers or possibly both of you are plagued by long work hours and stress.

It is too easy to dismiss stress as a normal working condition.

Chronic stress, as much as we do not want it, is our modern-day birthright.

Are there days when you feel that your stress is going to cause you to explode?

For many corporate warriors their everyday stress is out of control.

Stress is costly and that includes the productivity cost and the financial cost.

If you are the boss, you must wonder why more of your people have not just walked away from their jobs.

WORKPLACE STRESS AND PRODUCTIVITY LOSSES

Every day stress is impacting the health, performance, and productivity of corporate warriors.

In October of 2018, Korn Ferry conducted a survey of approximately 2,000 professionals which asked them about the impact of their workplace stress.

According to the survey, nearly 2/3 of the survey respondents say their stress levels at work are higher now than they were 5 years ago.

Some of the factors that have caused the increased stress levels at work include keeping up with the changes in technology, the increase in workloads and interpersonal conflict.

More than 3/4 of the survey respondents say stress at work has had a negative impact on their personal relationships, and 2/3 say they have lost sleep due to work stress.

16% say they've had to quit a job due to stress, a significant number.

35% of the respondents say their boss is their biggest source of stress at work.

80% say it is a change in leadership that impacts their level of stress.

Numerous other studies have shown that younger workers, women and those in lower-skilled jobs are at the most risk of experiencing work-related stress.

29% of workers reported feeling extreme stress because of their jobs according to a survey completed by Yale University.

This stress directly costs employers billions of dollars each year.

Job-related stress has escalated over the past few decades and is the major source of stress for American adults according to numerous studies.

The effects of job-related stress are evident in workers' physical health, mental health and their behavior.

Workplace stress contributes significantly to a decline in a company's overall success and this means lower profits.

Workers who are stressed at work are more likely to engage in unhealthy behaviors, such as cigarette smoking, alcohol and drug abuse and poor dietary patterns.

Now more than ever, it is important to take proactive measures to prevent stress by either removing or reducing the potential stressors of any and all types.

Workplace stress is manageable, and you must address this stress before it takes control of you, your employees and your business.

RESPOND TO YOUR STRESS

Stress is real, and for some of us it is always there.

Stress is a killer.

Stress is a normal part of life and you can experience stress from both inside and outside influences.

Some of us are much better at responding to our stress than others.

Is this you?

You were not hardwired to respond to your stress in the best possible way.

Let me elaborate. Your primitive 500-year-old brain is not hardwired for response.

Even though we have evolved as humans, a lot of our behavior is still dictated by our prehistoric brain, not by our modern evolved brain.

Our non-evolved brains are also known as the reptilian brain or the lizard brain. And there's only one thing our prehistoric brain is concerned with.

Responding to survive, and that does not always mean the response was well thought out.

When the stress is overwhelming you can choose to respond in one of three ways:

1. Fight

2. Flight

3. Or choose to respond appropriately

You must take 100% responsibility and respond to your stress.

There are no excuses for anything less.

When it comes to thinking about survival, a lot of it is black and white.

Whatever you are dealing with, it is not always easy to figure out what your next step should be.

However, there are things that you can do to reduce your stress. When life takes those unexpected turns, you must respond appropriately.

Start responding now.

While some stress is easy to respond to ourselves, at times it helps to have someone hold your hand and help you navigate through the rough waters of stress.

That is exactly what I want to do for you.

As a Canfield Trainer, someone that trains individuals in the "The Success Principles" I have a deep understanding of Principle Number One and utilize this principal as a guide in dealing with my stress.

Principle number one is revealed in this formula:

$$E+R=O$$

EVENT + RESPONSE = OUTCOME

- EVENTS are what happen to us.

- RESPONSES are how we respond to these events.

- OUTCOMES are the result of our responses to those events.

Everything you do is a result of your choices. Your outcome is up to you.

You must also respond to your stress the right way.

The question that I have for you is:

Are you interested in enjoying the benefits from responding to your stress instead of reacting?

THE STRESS SOLUTION

The stress solution is not medication, and it is not alcohol.

The stress solution is meditation, and meditation needs to be taught to those that work in the highly stressful corporate world.

We have reached a tipping point, and you need to utilize meditation as part of your wellness strategy.

Your employees and your profits are counting on it.

When you learn to meditate, you will be able to reduce your stress, increase your inner calmness and clarity and be happier.

Meditation is the best investment that you can make to facilitate a stress-reduced workplace.

Your profits are counting on it.

WHAT IS MEDITATION?

When you hear the word meditation, what do you think of?

Meditation is defined as a practice where an individual uses a technique, such as focusing their mind on an object, thought or activity, to achieve a mentally clear and emotionally calm state.

The history of meditation is very long and rich. As its benefits became more well known, it has grown in popularity.

Today, meditation is an important activity in the lives of millions of people worldwide, and meditation can be practiced by anyone.

Meditation is endorsed by many doctors as it is known to have many health benefits.

This former corporate warrior created Easy to Meditate as an easy way to learn how to meditate, after hundreds of hours of studying and practicing meditation.

Easy to Meditate can be easily learned and practiced by anyone and I can help you to create a daily meditation practice that will change your life.

So why should corporate warriors meditate?

WHY YOU SHOULD MEDITATE

Meditation has more than one hundred benefits and it has become a part of the daily lives of many corporate warriors.

Meditating for even short periods of time can have positive benefits.

Meditation can help you learn how to navigate your stress storms and can help you maintain both your physical and your mental health.

With a daily meditation practice, you will be more relaxed, your mind will be clearer, and your body will be healthier.

With Easy to Meditate, you can change the way that your brain processes information and the way that your sympathetic nervous system responds to stress.

Utilizing Easy to Meditate will help you decrease your stress levels, and this will lead to better long-term health, wellness and happiness.

A regular meditation practice utilizing Easy to Meditate changes your brain in ways that can help you to control your emotions, enhance your concentration, decrease your stress and even become more connected to those around you.

The benefits that are available with Easy to Meditate are available to anyone who makes time to develop a meditation practice.

The goal of Easy to Meditate is not to control your thoughts. Easy to Meditate allows you to reach a new level of inner calm.

The biggest benefit of Easy to Meditate is that it will help you reduce the stress that can wear you out both mentally and physically because when people get stressed, their minds go into overdrive.

Easy to Meditate can pump the breaks on this response.

Over the past decade a consensus has emerged from the medical community that shows that chronic stress causes numerous problems including high blood pressure, decreased immunity and impaired cognitive functions.

According to a 2013 study by the journal, Health Psychology, the practice of meditation was shown to have an impact on the reduction of cortisol, the stress hormone.

The study followed its participants for three months, and their cortisol levels were measured both before and after the study. The study found that cortisol levels trended downward.

Mental clutter is the junk that not only takes up space in our heads, but it continues to live there rent-free, and the rent is due every day.

Our mental clutter sends us on all sorts of twists and turns and eventually leads us down a road that goes nowhere fast.

If you let it, your mental clutter will move in and take permanent residence in your mind.

Easy to Meditate helps you get rid of your mental clutter. Stop being a mental hoarder, and let it go.

Opioids are pain-reducing chemicals that you can take as pain-relieving medications to flood your brain with these chemicals. These drugs can have devastating side effects. Meditation, utilizing Easy to Meditate, can help you to reduce pain without releasing these chemicals.

A 2016 study found that a meditation practice can significantly reduce the intensity of pain and its unpleasantness in the body.

The Journal of Neuroscience reports that you can save a lot of money on prescription drug costs, while simultaneously relieving pain more effectively, by using meditation.

As someone who takes more than a few drugs for multiple sclerosis, I can tell you personally that medications can have bothersome side effects.

This is not true with Easy to Meditate. There is no pain, addiction or any side effects.

None.

Hypertension, also known as high blood pressure, can be a deadly condition, and keeping your blood pressure in check is critical for maintaining good health and the prevention of heart attacks, strokes and heart disease.

Dr. Randy Zusman at Massachusetts General Hospital explained to National Public Radio (NPR) how prescribing meditation for patients with high blood pressure could lead to a reduction in need for common blood pressure medication.

Meditation can help elicit the "relaxation response" and when you are relaxed, nitric oxide produced by your body helps blood vessels open. This helps to reduce blood pressure.

When patients are taught to meditate in order to achieve the relaxation response, the results have been very encouraging.

More than 60% of patients found that the relaxation response helped to lower their blood pressure.

Dr. Randy Zusman stated that blood pressure was lowered for some patients to the point of enabling them to stop taking some of their medication.

Research has shown that meditation can also help you with your self-control.

Depression is like the plague. Doctors and scientists have been searching for a cure that doesn't come with the side effects.

Depression affects about 20% of adults ages 65 and older and can lead to higher risks for heart disease and death from illnesses. Depression also makes 's people feel more socially isolated.

Some doctors have found that depression can be alleviated with a daily meditation practice. Meditation has also been found to change regions of the brain that are specifically linked with depression.

Another way meditation helps the brain is by protecting the hippocampus or the brain area involved in memory.

Your immune system is a complex group of processes in your body that fight infection and disease and a vigorous immune system is crucial to living a healthy life.

Stress plays havoc with your immune system, and this means that you are more likely to become sick.

Several recent studies have shown that meditation can play an important role in maintaining and even strengthening your immune system. New studies are coming out on a regular basis probing the positive impact that meditation has on the complex immune system.

New studies are coming out on a regular basis probing the positive impact that meditation and your ability to develop a calmness, and this can help you to communicate more effectively.

According to researchers at the Infanta Cristina Hospital in Spain, meditation was shown to increase the level of cells in our blood that fight off viruses and bacteria.

Another study done at UCLA found that meditation in older adults can prevent the expression of a certain group of genes that activate inflammation.

Easy to Meditate is simple, relaxing, and you don't have to join a religion or a cult.

All over the world meditators report that they are happier since starting their meditation practice because it reduces stress that is caused by our hectic, multi-tasking lives.

For example, if a co-worker, supervisor or anyone else yells at you, what is your natural first reaction?

Do you yell back, become silent, or at the very least, become defensive?

Do you blame others instead of walking away or taking a step back and taking responsibility for your part in the argument?

When you meditate, clinical studies from UCLA have shown that you are able to think more rationally and logically.

For people with chronic pain, meditation can help reduce the amount of medicine that is needed (remember to always check with your medical provider) and in some cases eliminate or at least reduce medication.

This is great news for those that have problems with medications and the effects.

After a double discectomy (back surgery), I eliminated all pain medication within 48 hours.

Harvard Health reports that meditation can help fight insomnia. Meditation can help you fall asleep more easily and sleep more soundly.

Many meditators experience better sleep, including me.

Some people find a period of meditation before bed is helpful, but studies have shown that a meditation practice at any point during the day benefits our sleeping habits.

The benefits of meditation are an asset to corporate warriors.

Meditation can also be beneficial to those that will be interviewing for a new job or position. Meditation can help with the apprehension and panic.

Concentration can evade us when we need it the most, and for some corporate warriors, concentration is a problem.

Meditation helps because it can increase the ability to concentrate and focus and can encourage creativity, promote problem-solving skills and decrease the stress associated with multitasking.

In this chapter, we have discussed some of the many benefits of a regular meditation practice for the corporate warrior.

We each have our own reason or reasons for developing our own meditation practice, and it is easy to develop a meditation utilizing Easy to Meditate.

MEDITATION MYTHS AND TRUTHS

Here are some of the myths surrounding meditation.

Myth-Meditation and Mindfulness are the same thing.

Truth-While the terms are sometimes used interchangeably, meditation and mindfulness are not the same thing.

Mindfulness is maintaining an awareness of your thoughts, feelings, bodily sensations, and surrounding environment, through a gentle, nurturing personal lens.

Meditation is a practice where an individual uses a technique, such as focusing their mind on an object, thought or activity, to achieve a clear and emotionally calm state.

Myth-Meditation can only be practiced by religious people or gurus.

Truth- My meditation technique is called Easy to Meditate for a reason. Meditation can be practiced by anyone and everyone.

Myth-Meditating is complicated.

Truth-Meditation is actually a simple practice and can be practiced by anyone, including children.

You don't need to develop a practice where you meditate 5 times a day in places that are non-conducive to meditating to enjoy the benefits.

You can start meditating with 3 to 5 minutes a day and build on it. Meditation does not take a lot of time. Your meditation practice is up to you.

Myth- Meditation will turn you into someone that you are not.

Truth-Meditation helps to eliminate mental clutter and facilitate inner peace. It lets the best of who you are come to the surface.

Myth-Meditation makes you zone out and makes your mind go blank.

Truth-Meditation does not stop you from thinking. It does not make your mind go blank and it does not zone you out. Rather, it is calming and relaxing.

Myth-Meditation puts you into an altered state where the mind is completely empty of thoughts.

Truth-Easy to Meditate is about quieting your mind and your body. There is no trance involved.

Myth-You must become a Buddhist or take up some other type of religion.

Truth –I am a Jewish guy from New York, the farthest thing from a Buddhist.

Meditation does not discriminate nor require you to convert or follow any religion.

THE TRUTH ABOUT
EASY TO MEDITATE

Everyone can benefit from a daily meditation practice.

Now that you have read the previous chapters of this book, it is time to ask yourself:

- How can I personally benefit from a daily meditation practice?

- What would my cost be for not creating a daily meditation practice?

- What is the cost of maintaining the status quo and doing nothing?

I am very grateful that I did ask myself those questions, and I am sure that you will be grateful too.

I had known of meditation, but I knew nothing specifically about it.

But after jumping in to adopt a daily meditation practice myself, I can assure you that it will change your life for the better.

Before I began my daily practice of meditation, my stress levels could reach a 20 on a 1 to 10 scale.

Not good for me. Not good for anyone.

Now while I am still affected by stress, it is very different.

For millions, including me, meditation has been a life changer. It has helped me to relax, de-stress and to find a new calm.

The questions that I have for you are:

Are you interested in reducing your stress?

Are you interested in a calmer mind?

Are you interested in fighting off stress and anxiety-related sickness?

Are you committed to taking an easy and simple action daily to benefit yourself?

If you are, then follow me.

WHEN SHOULD YOU MEDITATE?

Before recommending the best time of day to meditate, it is important to be clear that you can meditate at any time of the day or night.

When you wake up, your brain is still quiet, so why not prime the pumps first?

Meditation is to your mind what yoga and exercise is to your body.

Whether you feel it or not, your meditation practice will support you all day long.

How is that?

Meditation provides you space from the manic nature of your mind.

In the morning, nearly everyone is still asleep. There is quiet and peace, and that early morning peace and quiet has a very positive effect.

There are usually no distractions, and meditation is an incredibly powerful way to start the day.

When you meditate soon after you get up in the morning, it means that you are putting yourself first.

Meditation is a very powerful expression of self-care that will have all sorts of positive effects, and if you do this regularly, you will strengthen and build your practice.

Meditation can bring you clarity and ease.

When you enter your day having meditated, you feel good. It's amazing what this can do for your outlook on the day. You can meditate at other times in the day though.

I recommend that you follow my advice and meditate in the morning.

When you do this, you will carry that peace with you into your day.

HOW TO MEDITATE

Over the years, lots of people have asked my advice on how to start their meditation practice.

This eventually led to the creation of my signature system, Easy to Meditate.

Easy to Meditate was designed to be done in any comfortable place that you prefer, including your office.

Here is my easy step by step approach. But, first a bit of insight.

If you are new to meditation, it's important to remember to be easy on yourself. The idea is to reduce your stress, not to add to it. Exhale and let your stress go.

When your start meditating you may have relaxing experiences right away, or it may take days, weeks or even months.

Personally, while I started feeling a sense of calm right away, it took a few weeks to develop my daily practice, my meditation habit and to really feel the benefits of my practice.

Originally, I imagined myself sitting quietly with my legs crossed, dressed like a monk when I first inquired about and learned how to meditate.

Meditation for the beginner can seem daunting and perceived as dull.

Not with Easy to Meditate though.

I believe in an easy and safe meditation practice. That is why I created this super simple way to meditate that anyone can use.

And I just don't believe in getting hurt when meditating, whether it be by falling, walking into traffic, falling off a ledge or down the stairs.

It makes absolutely no sense to have a dangerous meditation practice. That means no walking meditation and no dancing meditation. No roadside meditating either.

Ok?

Getting started learning to meditate using Easy to Meditate is quite easy.

If it was difficult, then it might just add more stress to your life, and that is something that you do not want.

You learn to meditate, by meditating.

The silence and the diminished stress you will experience when you meditate are so attractive and welcome, that as time goes on, you will naturally want to meditate for longer periods of time.

Here is my step by step approach.

1. Choose a nice, quiet and comfortable place where you won't be disturbed for 3 to 20 minutes or longer. A place that you are comfortable with will make it easier for you to meditate.

2. Make sure to find a spot that's relatively quiet where you'll be undisturbed.

3. Dress comfortably. Nothing tight and nothing restrictive.

4. Sit in a comfortable place with your back straight. Relax and rest your hands on your lap. Sit quietly and close your eyes or focus on an object in front of you.

5. Take a minute or two to settle yourself.

6. You can sit on the floor with the support of a meditation cushion or on any chair with your feet resting on the ground. It is not necessary to force yourself into any position if it is not comfortable.

7. Regardless of how you sit, it is important to maintain the natural curve of your back. That means no slouching. If you have chronic back problems and cannot sit for a prolonged period, try another position.

8. Sit quietly with your eyes closed, exhale and relax your muscles.

9. Thoughts will come. Just sit silently in an effortless way.

10. Close your eyes gently and breathe slowly, deeply and gently. Begin by taking a few slow and deep breaths, inhaling with your nose and exhaling from your mouth. Don't force your breathing. Let it come naturally.

11. Your first few breaths of air are likely to be shallow, but as you allow more air to fill your lungs each time, your breaths will gradually become deeper and fuller.

12. Focus your attention on your breathing. Continue to focus on your breath for as long as you like. Take as long as you need and breathe slowly and deeply.

13. If you find your attention straying away from your breaths, just gently bring it back. It may happen many times.

14. Each time you catch your mind wandering during the counting, and it absolutely will, bring

your attention back to your breathing and start over again.

15. Everyone experiences this during meditation no matter how long they have been practicing.

16. Everyone who meditates goes through periods where we start feeling that inner stress or crazy but stick with it.

17. It is referred to by some as "monkey mind." I don't know a single person that meditates that has not gone through it.

18. Just stick with it.

19. This can sometimes be easier said than done. Getting your mind to cooperate can be like house training a new puppy.

20. It is not easy, but it can be done. Don't give up. Stick with it.

21. When you are ready to end your meditation session, open your eyes and stand up slowly. Stretch yourself.

22. Well done! You have done it!

23. Initially, start meditating every morning for 3–20 minutes and every evening for 3–20 minutes.

24. The most important thing when you start meditating is to just start and to be committed.

25. Create a habit and stick with it. This means committing to meditate every day, and to make meditation a regular practice. No exceptions, no excuses, no "not today."

Meditation does not require any special equipment or clothes. It does not require that you go on any pricey retreat.

If you commit 100% to meditating daily, you will see the results.

Be committed and be disciplined.

The benefits are there for you to realize, but you must do the work.

CREATING YOUR MEDITATION HABIT

Learning to meditate is not difficult, but it takes commitment. You need a simple and easy protocol for the creation of your meditation habit.

In order to realize the benefits of meditation, you must practice it regularly and consistently.

In 2010, a study conducted at University College London showed that it takes an average of 66 days to build a new habit. This means that you need to consistently spend about two months creating your meditation habit.

You can meditate during the morning, day, or night or at any time when you feel the need to calm down, reset or just get balanced.

I suggest that you pick a regular time that you can set aside every day to meditate. In order to help you set the habit it is important to have a reminder or a trigger that reminds you to perform your meditation practice every day.

I have found that the easiest way to do this is to incorporate meditation into your morning routine before your day gets busy.

For many that I have spoken with, first thing in the morning is best. Get your day started off right.

This is not a must. You can meditate any time of day. I suggest that you do not meditate right before bed. The reason is that too many people fall asleep, and while I am not someone that is against sleep, the point of meditation is to meditate, not sleep. This is important so that you can achieve the benefits of meditation.

Remember that meditation is not and should not feel like a job; it is a lifestyle choice.

Meditating for just 5 to 10 minutes a day has been shown to have a positive impact. Meditating for 20 minutes or longer has shown to have even more benefits, so preferably you would meditate for 20 minutes or longer every day.

Some days you may have a limited amount of time, and therefore, you cannot meditate for the same length of time. The key is to keep at it and meditate every day.

You may experience times where you do not feel like it pays to continue meditating. This happens. Stay with your practice though. Consistency is the key when developing your meditation practice.

The key to creating consistency is to find a place that you are comfortable with. A place that resonates with you and one that you can make your meditation spot.

Decide on a length of time that you will commit to every day. As I have previously said, start meditating every morn-ing for 3–20 minutes and if possible, every evening for 3–20 minutes.

A meditation practice is like brushing your teeth. You need to be consistent and do it every day.

Track your progress and stay accountable. Use the Easy to Meditate journal. One of the bonuses for purchasing this book is a week long journal that you should utilize to journal and track your meditation practice. Using the Easy to Meditate journal will help you track your prog-ress. When you use the journal and track your prog-ress it is more difficult to skip a day. With smartphones there are habit tracking apps available. Choose one and use one if you prefer this way of tracking.

There is also a 66-day version that you can use that is available for a small investment.

There is an old saying "Whatever gets rewarded, gets repeated". To help get your meditation habit to stick, reward yourself. It can be as simple as giving yourself a pat on the back or a drink like a cup of coffee or an iced tea.

Another method of creating a meditation habit is to have an accountability. Some of my students have been couples and when there is someone that holds you accountable, you will find it easier to create a meditation habit and more difficult to skip a meditation session. Accountability partner matters.

Consistent action is the only way to create and make meditation a regular habit. Practice meditation every day and create an automatic habit. When you make meditation a long-term habit it will transform your life.

FREQUENTLY ASKED QUESTIONS

Q: How often should I utilize Easy to Meditate?

A: Ideally you will develop a meditation practice in which you meditate once a day, or possibly twice a day.

Some people prefer to meditate in the morning before breakfast and have another session later in the day or evening.

At first, meditation may seem like a job, but you will learn to enjoy it and look forward to it every day.

View your meditation practice as an opportunity to relax your mind rather than an item on your to-do list. It is an opportunity to spend some quiet time with yourself.

Cultivate meditation as a habit that you'd do naturally every day, like brushing of your teeth.

Q: How long do I need to meditate each time?

A: Aim to meditate for at least 3 minutes to start and 15 minutes or more for each session once you get started.

For most people, it will normally take 3 to 5 minutes or more for the mind to settle down. If your meditation is too short, you might find the session has ended before you even have a chance to get into it.

Q. Should I use a timer?

A: If you want to. It is ok to periodically glance at a clock or watch but train your body and mind to meditate for your desired time period until it becomes second nature.

There are several meditation apps available for your phone and other timers available for a small investment.

Q: Why do I find it so hard to concentrate or sit still during Easy to Meditate?

A: Many people, including experienced long-time meditators, experience occasions when they find their concentration is not as focused as they want it to be.

It is important to be patient with yourself, especially if you are a beginner. Meditation helps you calm your mind, but it may not start out that way. If you find yourself having a hard time sitting still during meditation, try to avoid going anything that stimulates your mind just before you start meditating because it is not going to be very helpful.

Some people also find stretching before meditation helps them to get into a relaxed state faster.

Q: When I meditate, I feel like I'm betraying my religious beliefs. Why is that?

A: This is a common myth. Meditation is often associated with foreign cultures and religions, such as Buddhism, because that is where it originated.

That is why many people have mistakenly equated meditation with a religion when in it is not.

On the other hand, some forms of meditation do involve the visualization of popular religious icons or repeating of mantras from religious texts.

Labeling meditation as religious just because of its diverse use is as good as saying all knives are weapons of destruction and hence should be avoided.

While it is true that some religions include meditation as part of their observance, Easy to Meditate is not religious.

Though it may not be apparent to you, there is a transformation taking place within you every time you meditate. The process is slow, but it is happening.

Q: Should I close my eyes?

A: Closing your eyes is optional, but I recommend it. It is not necessary to close your eyes while doing meditation.

Meditating with your eyes opened or closed is a personal preference. You should experiment to see what feels comfortable and gives you the best results.

Q: What should I wear when meditating?

A: While there is no specific dress code for meditation, I recommend that you wear something nonrestrictive and comfortable.

Always be comfortable.

Q: What should I do if I feel like I am going to fall asleep during meditation?

A: Allowing more light to enter the eyes is a good way to stay awake. Lifting your eyelids higher, while keeping your gaze soft and unfocused, will help to keep the brain stimulated and alert. Your physical and mental states also play a key role.

When you are lethargic, it is much harder to concentrate, which means you will need to put in more effort to stay awake. Accept it and remind yourself to keep at it.

Q: How do I know I'm meditating?

A: When you are focused on your breathing, yet fully aware of the random thoughts in your mind and not distracted by them you are meditating.

Q; Do I need a teacher to learn how to meditate?

A: No, you do not, but I do recommend that you take advantage of what you learn here and visit www.Easy-ToMeditate.com to join our supportive community.

WHAT TO EXPECT WITH EASY TO MEDITATE?

Based on my experience, there are a few things to expect when you utilize Easy to Meditate to learn how to meditate.

Do not worry. It is nothing funky or weird. It is just the opposite. You may feel blank, like nothing is happening.

This is good. That sense of calm and stillness is something that you should strive for.

Then there is something referred to as "monkey mind".

Monkey mind will not hurt you, and it will not ruin your day. Your mind feels like it is going in different directions. Monkey mind is different for everyone.

Don't be surprised by the sudden urges that you will get. Some of these urges will include:

- Getting up

- Putting on the television or radio

- Eating

- And a lot more

Resist these urges and keep meditating.

These and other urges happen to everyone at one time or another, to both new to more experienced meditators.

STAYING MOTIVATED
TO MEDITATE

Easy to Meditate is a habit that is worth starting and sticking with because there are many benefits associated with a regular Easy to Meditate meditation practice.

Easy to Meditate has a weeklong Meditation Challenge. Visit www.EasyToMeditate.com to sign up.

The Easy to Meditate meditation Challenge will provide you the foundation for a regular practice.

It will be a momentum builder for the rest of your life.

Find out about the challenge at www.EasyToMeditate. com

CONCLUSION

This simple beginner's manual for Easy to Meditate will help you start and Easy to Meditate practice and it can help you become a better meditator if you already have a meditation practice.

You will find inspiration for your daily practice when you become a part of the supportive Easy to Meditate community. Join the community at www.EasyToMeditate.com and receive support, read informative blog posts and watch snackable videos that are designed just for you.

You will find the solutions to your struggles when you become a part of the supportive Easy to Meditate community.

You will find in-depth answers to your questions about meditation when you become a part of the supportive Easy to Meditate community.

If you become a part of the Easy to Meditate community you will not be sorry, and you will not look back.

Developing an Easy to Meditate meditation practice has changed my life and the lives of others. It can change your life too.

I know that it can feel difficult at first but meditating regularly utilizing the Easy to Meditate technique will be one of the best things that you could do for yourself.

Easy to Meditate will change your life and the lives of those around you.

Easy to Meditate is the one thing that you can do to benefit your mind and your body on both on a short and long-term basis.

Give Easy to Mediate a chance and you will not look back.

EASY TO MEDITATE EXTRAS

For FREE resources that are available for readers of this book, visit the resources page at www.EasyToMeditate.com and enter your email address.

THANK YOU FROM ADAM WEBER

Thank you for reading this short book "Easy to Meditate."

As you develop your meditation practice utilizing the Easy to Meditate technique, you will enjoy the benefits and rewards discussed here.

This book is your one-stop entry point for creating and practicing meditation daily.

No experience or skills required.

Creating a meditation practice is not rocket science, but it is something that some people stumble with when lacking a little bit of guidance or hand holding.

You need a guide who can show you how it is done the RIGHT way. (And there are lots of "wrong ways" to learn to develop a meditation habit.)

Just reading this short book will put you miles ahead of most people that try to develop a meditation habit without the right guidance.

Do not overthink this.

Visit www.EasyToMeditate.com and contact me.

Welcome to the Easy to Meditate community.

Adam

BONUS CHAPTERS

YOUR TO DO LIST

To do lists are popular for some, even necessary for others. We have all had them, and they need no introduction.

It's easy to see why these lists are so popular. You list the items that you need to get done on a piece of paper or a device, like your smart phone. You then check off the boxes or cross items off the list as they are done.

Do you have a to-do list?

How about a not-to-do list?

Some productivity experts say a not to do list is as if not more important than a to-do list.

What is a not-to-do list?

It is a list of things that you absolutely should not do. These tasks don't move you toward any of your larger objectives. They are not necessary for you to do.

You are much better off not doing them. They should either be left undone or you should delegate them to someone else.

The most successful people that I know say that wonderful things arise when you learn to say no.

Our time and energy are limited resources and for each of us and how we choose to spend those precious resources matters a lot.

Your not-to-do list will bring you clarity and inner peace. It will also bring you greater transparency and improve your relationships with others by not making promises you can't keep.

BREATHE

Breathe, before your stress surfaces, not just when your stress surfaces.

When stress surfaces, your breathing rate and your breathing patterns change.

Are you starting to feel stressed or anxious?

Stop and take a few breaths.

When you are stressed, instead of breathing slowly from your lower lungs, you breathe rapidly and shallowly from your upper lungs.

Breathing rapidly can cause you to hyperventilate and in turn this can explain your uncomfortable symptoms during panic.

Deep breathing is called diaphragmatic breathing, abdominal breathing, belly breathing, and paced respiration.

When you breathe deeply, the air coming in through your nose fully fills your lungs, and your lower belly rises. For some, deep breathing seems unnatural.

With deep abdominal breathing you feel incoming oxygen and outgoing carbon dioxide.

This can slow your heartbeat and lower or stabilize your blood pressure.

Preferably, focus on slow, and deep breathing.

First, find a quiet, comfortable place to sit or lie down. Then take a normal breath, and then try a deep breath: Breathe in slowly through your nose, allowing your chest and lower belly to rise as you fill your lungs. Let your abdomen expand fully. Now breathe out slowly through your mouth or your nose, if that feels more natural.

As you sit comfortably with your eyes closed, blend deep breathing with helpful imagery and perhaps a focus word or phrase that helps you relax. An example of this would be to breathe slowly and count backwards from 10 to 1.

Several techniques can help you change your response to stress and you may want to try different relaxation techniques to see which one works best for you.

You may want to try the following two steps.

1. Choose a place where you can sit or lie down
    comfortably and quietly.

2. Don't try too hard. Just breathe. Breathing too
    hard may just cause you to tense up.

The key to eliciting your relaxation response lies in shift-
ing your focus from stress to deep and calm rhythms.

In order to establish a habit always practice at the same
time. Practice once or twice a day and try to practice at
least 10 minutes each day.

The following is a breathing exercise modeled after "box
breathing".

It is a powerful relaxation tool that can help clear your
mind, relax your body, and allow you to focus.

1. Close your eyes. Breathe in through your nose,
    slowly counting to four. Feel the air filling your
    lungs.

2. Hold your breath here and slowly count to four
    again. Try not to clamp your airway shut. Simply
    avoid inhaling or exhaling for four counts.

3. Slowly exhale to the count of four.

4. Hold the exhale for another four count.

5. Repeat steps 1–4 for 4 minutes or until you feel
    calm and centered.

VISUALIZATION

Visualization is one of the most powerful tools that you can utilize.

As you visualize a desired outcome regularly (preferably daily), and you believe that what you are visualizing is possible, your brain will increase your motivation to make it happen.

Visualization will help you become more determined to do what is necessary to achieve your goals and desires and you will become more motivated.

In addition to your increased motivation, you will begin to get ideas that will help you to achieve your goals and desires.

You may wake up in the middle of the night with a brilliant idea, thought or even experience a moment of pure genius while you are in the shower or out for a run.

This happens because visualization prompts your brain to "wake up" to messages and resources that it previously shut out. Now that it is aware of your goal, it will assist you in becoming more aware to finding the answers and a path to achieving that goal. Your brain will assist you.

For visualization to work, you need to have a crystal-clear clear vision of what you want.

Envision what you would like what you want to see happen in your life.

Do you want to buy a new house?

Do you want to be married to the man or woman of your dreams?

Are you getting the idea?

Early in his career, Jack Canfield, best-selling author of the Success Principles and a champion of high performance and achieving success, had never earned more than $8,000 in a year. When he began to visualize daily and focused on the goal of earning $100,000 in a year, he began to come up with ideas as to how to achieve this breakthrough after only 30 days.

According to Jack, these ideas were always with him, but it just took visualization to make them come to the surface.

As he began to program his mind through visualization, his brain found the ways to earn $100,000. Jack was able to achieve this goal in less than one year and has continued to increase his income and success over the years.

Jack said, "Your brain wants to solve your problems". " When you get 'stuck' it simply means that your mind isn't open to the solutions.

Visualization releases this resistance and allows the brain to do its job and make you happy."

To visualize, use the following six steps to incorporate visualization into your daily routine.

Step 1. You must first decide exactly what you want. Be very clear about it.

Step 2. Choose at least one image to hold in your mind's eye as you go through your visualization process.

Step 3. Get comfortable and focus on relaxing and your breathing.

Step 4. Visualize the image daily. Begin visualization in a private place where you will be undisturbed, a place that is quiet and shut off from the world if possible.

Step 5. Visualize the steps that you will take and OR on the specific goal, or success that you are reaching for

Step 6. Walk through it like a movie, and not just still images. Focus on achieving success Step into the feeling and power of this image; make it very real.

Start out by visualizing for 5 minutes each day for a week and then increase how long that you visualize each day, each week and going forward.

STAY HYDRATED

Fatigue, dizziness and confusion are just a few of the unpleasant signs that you may be dehydrated. To avoid them, you must keep up with proper fluid intake.

Most people do not drink enough water. When you drink enough water, your body is hydrated. You can flush your body of toxic substances and improve your body's ability to perform its vital functions.

"We lose water every day through natural bodily functions, but dehydration occurs when we lose more bodily fluids than we're taking in," says Jennifer Williams, MPH, a Columbus, Ohio based nutrition scientist and hydration expert at Abbott Laboratories. "Because humans are made up of mostly water and electrolytes, we need to maintain the proper balance of these in our system."

Being dehydrated impairs your body's ability to perform its vital functions.

Staying hydrated will not only help you avoid dehydrations negative side effects, but it will help you feel better overall by improving your mood, boosting brain function, and preventing fatigue, Williams says.

Becoming dehydrated generally doesn't sneak up on you. There are physical signs of dehydration, including headaches, fatigue, vomiting, and a flushed complexion, he says.

You may also feel more irritable and like your energy has been zapped, says Sean Hashmi, MD, regional physician director of weight management and clinical nutrition for Kaiser Permanente in Woodland Hills, California.

Dr. Hashmi says, "The body is such an incredible machine that it has built-in mechanisms that allow you to know when you need more or less water".

Your body needs water to survive. Every cell, tissue, and every organ in your body needs water to work properly.

Water helps your body use water to maintain its temperature, remove waste, and lubricate your joints. You should drink water every day. Water is needed for overall good health.

Most people have been told that they should drink 6 to 8, 8-ounce glasses of water each day. While that seems like a reasonable goal, different people need different amounts of water to stay hydrated.

Some people can stay well hydrated by just drinking whenever they feel thirsty. Others may need fluids each day.

If you are concerned that you are not drinking enough water, look at your urine. If your urine is usually colorless or light yellow, you are likely well hydrated. If your urine is a dark yellow or amber color, you may be dehydrated.

Water is better for staying hydrated than many of the other alternative choices.

While some drinks and foods can help you stay hydrated, they may also add extra calories, sugar and other chemicals to your diet.

Fruit and vegetable juices, milk, and herbal teas can add to the amount of water you get each day but are not perfect choices for all people.

Even caffeinated drinks like, coffee, tea, and soda can contribute to your daily water intake.

Strike that. Stop drinking soda. It is rotting your body, from the inside out.

The more research that is done, the more that we are finding out that energy or sports drinks are not that good for you. Most of these drinks are high in added sugar and other preservatives.

Actively prevent dehydration by drinking plenty of water. Don't wait until you notice symptoms of dehydration to drink and stay hydrated.

Some people are at higher risk of dehydration, including people who exercise at a high intensity or in hot weather for too long, have certain medical conditions (such as kidney stones, bladder infection), are sick (fever, vomiting, diarrhea), are pregnant or breastfeeding, are trying to lose weight, or are not able to get enough fluids during the day. Older adults are also at higher risk. As you get older, your brain may not be able to sense dehydration. It doesn't send signals for thirst.

Water makes up more than half of your body weight. Every day you lose water when you go to the bathroom, sweat, and even when you breathe. You lose water even faster when the weather is hot, when you are physically active, or if you have a fever.

Vomiting and diarrhea can also lead to rapid water loss. If you don't replace the water you lose, you will become dehydrated.

EAT RIGHT

Eating right is easier said than done.

It doesn't have to be tough.

Make sure to watch your portion sizes and choose real foods such as fruits, vegetables, whole grains and lean meats over junk and non-nutritious foods.

While it was well intended, the food pyramid that we have historically seen in school cafeterias and doctor's offices is deceiving, out of date and has been debunked by some health care professionals because it is not accurate based on today's nutritional needs and the evolution of the growth and the manufacture of our food today.

We live in a world where whole and real foods have been and are increasingly being replaced with altered and processed foods and during their growth, refinement or packaging many of our foods have become full of chemicals of all sorts.

The processing of many of the foods we eat have made them into an edible form of poison.

According to a 2011 review of 34 studies in the "Journal of the American Dietetic Association." Eating balanced meals with fruits and vegetables and listening to your hunger and fullness cues can help you to eat correctly.

You must choose healthier food and drink choices. Smart eating means choosing the right foods.

If all you have time for is a quick bite to eat from the gas station or a drugstore, you are not likely choosing a healthy option.

According to Rebecca Clyde, M.S., R.D.N., C.D., blogger at Nourish Nutrition, "A weekly meal plan can help you eat better, and save money and time during the week"

You must pay attention and listen to your hunger and fullness cues because ignoring those cues can lead to overeating and making unhealthy food choices. Eating slowly will give you time to listen to your fullness signals and reduce food intake at meals.

According to a 2008 study in the "Journal of the American Dietetic Association." You should stop eating before you feel full to ensure that your body gets the right amount of food.

You should include fruits and vegetables with every meal when possible, and they must be the right fruits and vegetables.

Try eating more salads without the unhealthy dressings. Add vegetables onto your plate because eating more fruits and vegetables provides your body with more vitamins, minerals, antioxidants and fiber.

A 2004 study in the "International Journal of Obesity and Related Metabolic Disorders" concluded that women with the largest increase in fruit and vegetable intake over a 12-year period had a lower risk of becoming obese.

And stop drinking soda. Soda is not healthy. Drink water because it will quench your thirst and decrease your soda craving.

There are many ways to eat healthy and you can eat healthy in a way that works for you and your family. Healthy eating can fit all tastes and traditions and can be affordable, too.

Small changes add up fast and help you to eat right.

SLEEP

We cut back on our sleep for work, for family demands, or even to watch a good movie or television show.

Even one night with a lack of sleep can affect you. You are more likely to be in a bad mood, less productive at work, or even involved in a car accident.

If not getting enough sleep is a regular part of your routine, you may get sick or even die early.

Feeling tired or drowsy during the day is one symptom of not getting enough sleep.

Have you ever found yourself lying in bed in the middle of the night and staring at the ceiling? Your mind is bouncing and racing.

You look at the clock and it is flashing 2 AM. Not being able to sleep is weighing on you.

When you cannot sleep it affects every aspect of your days, your nights, your life.

It doesn't have to be this way

Research has proven that lack of sleep can result in heart disease, lower cognitive function, weight gain, mood swings, and can affect your sexual performance.

1 in 3 people is sleep deprived. 1 in 4 suffer from insomnia.

The lack of sleep is part of our modern-day health crisis and it affects every system in our body.

In short, it is an important key to optimal health.

Your healthy sleep-wake cycle begins with the smart choices that you make throughout the day.

Sleep is an important performance activity and just like sports having the right equipment matters.

Here are five important habits that you can utilize to improve your sleep:

1. Aim to go to bed at the same time each night and aim to get up at the same time each morning.

2. Make sure your bedroom is quiet, dark, relaxing, and that the room temperature is comfortable.

3.   Remove your electronic devices, including televisions, computers, and smart phones, from the bedroom.

4.   Avoid large meals, caffeine, and alcohol before bedtime.

5.   Getting exercise during the day can help you fall asleep more easily at night.

Getting enough sleep is important. Sleep.

WORK WITH ADAM

There are five easy ways to work with Adam. The following five options are available based on your needs.

1. Read this short book, and then figure it out on your own.

2. Visit www.EasyToMeditate.com, read/watch the blog/vlog, and then figure it out on your own.

3. Invest in the Easy to Meditate online program. One program license per person.

4. Bring Adam into your business for training, coaching and get a special online program and video coaching after the training.

5. Custom training by design based on your organization's needs.

Please visit www.EasyToMeditate.com for lots of bonuses and so that we can decide if working together is a good fit.

ABOUT ADAM WEBER

Adam is a former corporate warrior that left the corporate world to help others learn to deal with their stress through the creation of Easy to Meditate, his proprietary process that helps others learn to meditate through either in-person or online training.

Adam's personal experience with an overload of stress started during his manic childhood.

To learn more about Easy to Meditate, visit www.EasyToMeditate.com.

When you join the Easy to Meditate community, you will be joining a supportive community of likeminded people, and you will gain access to a variety of easy-to-consume articles and training.

Adam is a Certified Canfield Trainer in The Success Principles and works with a variety of small, medium and larger clients to help them achieve their desired results and to support organizations from top to bottom.

For more information about Adam's offerings, please contact him at adam@easytomeditate.com

READER BONUS

Please visit
www.EasyToMeditate.com
to sign up for the free Easy
to Meditate 66 Day
Meditation Challenge

www.EasyToMeditate.com